The 90-Day Metabolic Reset Tracker

Track Your Glucose, Weight, Sleep, and Blood Pressure — and Watch Your Health Change

Gia

Publisher: Rooted Hound Press
Vienna, New Jersey

ISBN: 978-1-969687-16-7

Printed in the United States of America

Health Disclaimer

This workbook is intended for educational and informational purposes only. It is not intended to diagnose, treat, cure, or prevent any medical condition.

The information provided in this book should not be considered medical advice. Always consult a qualified healthcare professional before making changes to your diet, exercise routine, medications, or health management practices.

The author and publisher assume no responsibility for any health outcomes that may result from the use of this workbook.

Contents

Introduction

Your Body Is Always Talking

Your body sends signals every day.

Your weight changes slightly. Your blood pressure rises or falls. Your fasting glucose reflects the metabolic decisions your body made overnight. Your resting heart rate reveals stress, recovery, and physical conditioning.

Most people never see these signals clearly.

They step on a scale occasionally. They visit the doctor once a year. They may hear that a number is "high" or "borderline."

But what they rarely see are the **patterns**.

Patterns are where understanding begins.

Your metabolism is not random. It responds to sleep, food timing, activity, hydration, stress, and many other daily habits. Small choices repeated consistently shape how your body regulates energy, blood sugar, and cardiovascular health.

Tracking these signals over time reveals those patterns.

This workbook was created to help you do exactly that.

Why Daily Tracking Works

When you track your metabolic signals daily, something important happens: trends begin to emerge.

You may notice:

- Your fasting glucose improves when you finish dinner earlier.
- Your resting heart rate drops after a few weeks of regular walking.
- Your sleep improves when your evening routine becomes more consistent.
- Your blood pressure responds to hydration, stress levels, and physical activity.

These patterns often remain invisible until they are written down and observed over time.

Daily tracking turns scattered information into **meaningful insight**.

The Goal of This Workbook

This workbook is designed to help you observe and understand several core signals of metabolic health, including:

- Weight
- Waist circumference
- Blood pressure
- Resting heart rate
- Fasting glucose
- Sleep duration
- Physical activity

You do not need to track every metric perfectly.

What matters most is **consistency**.

Over ninety days, your daily entries will begin to reveal patterns that help you better understand how your body responds to lifestyle choices.

Progress Happens Through Small Changes

Improving metabolic health rarely comes from one dramatic change.

Instead, it comes from many small decisions repeated consistently:

- walking after meals
- improving sleep habits
- adjusting meal timing
- increasing daily movement
- choosing whole foods more often

These changes accumulate over time.

As you track your metabolic signals, you may begin to see how even modest adjustments can improve your numbers.

This Workbook Is a Tool for Awareness

The purpose of this workbook is not perfection.

It is awareness.

By observing your body's signals with curiosity and consistency, you give yourself the opportunity to make informed decisions that support long-term health. Over the next ninety days, this tracker will help you build that awareness — one day at a time.

When you learn your metabolic patterns, you are better able to make practical decisions. You may begin to notice which habits support steadier energy, better sleep, healthier glucose readings, improved recovery, or more consistent weight trends. This kind of awareness can help you respond earlier, make gradual adjustments, and have more informed conversations with your healthcare provider when needed.

Understanding Metabolic Health

Why Tracking Matters

Metabolic health influences many aspects of how we feel and function each day.

Energy levels, body weight, cardiovascular health, and blood sugar regulation are all connected to the body's metabolic systems. When these systems function well, the body maintains balance more easily. When they begin to drift out of balance, subtle warning signs often appear long before serious health problems develop.

These warning signs frequently show up in everyday numbers such as blood pressure, fasting glucose, resting heart rate, and waist circumference.

Unfortunately, many people only encounter these numbers during occasional medical visits. A single reading during a doctor's appointment offers only a snapshot of what is happening in that moment.

Metabolic health, however, changes gradually and responds continuously to daily habits.

Sleep quality, physical activity, stress levels, hydration, and food choices all influence the body's internal regulation systems. These influences accumulate day after day.

Tracking these signals regularly provides a clearer picture of how the body responds to those influences.

Over time, patterns become visible.

A person who records their fasting glucose may notice that late evening meals affect morning readings. Someone who tracks sleep alongside resting heart rate may observe how recovery improves with consistent rest.

These kinds of insights are difficult to see without written records.

Tracking transforms scattered information into meaningful data that reflects the body's ongoing metabolic story.

For many people, the act of recording these numbers also encourages greater awareness of daily habits. When progress becomes visible on paper, motivation often follows naturally.

Small improvements become visible and can be reinforced.

This workbook is designed to make that process simple.

By tracking several key metabolic signals consistently over ninety days, you create an opportunity to observe how your body responds to the choices you make each day.

Those observations can become the foundation for meaningful improvements in long-term health.

How to Use This Tracker

Recording Your Daily Metabolic Signals

Each row in the tracking table represents one day. Record your numbers as consistently as possible, ideally at the same time each day.

You do not need to track perfectly. The goal is to observe patterns over time, not to create perfect records.

What to Record in Each Column

Date

Write the calendar date.

Example:

3/12 or March 12

Weight

Record your body weight.

For best consistency:

• weigh yourself at the same time each day

• many people prefer first thing in the morning

Weight naturally fluctuates from day to day, so focus on long-term trends rather than daily changes.

Waist

Measure your waist circumference.

Tips for accurate measurement:

- measure at the same location each time
- many people measure just above the navel
- measure before eating if possible

Waist circumference can be a useful indicator of changes in abdominal fat and metabolic health.

BP (Blood Pressure)

Record your blood pressure reading.

Example format:

120 / 80

Tips for measuring blood pressure:

- sit quietly for 5 minutes before measuring
- keep your feet flat on the floor
- measure at roughly the same time each day

If you measure multiple readings, record the average.

HR (Resting Heart Rate)

Record your resting heart rate in beats per minute.

This can be measured:

- immediately after waking
- using a fitness tracker
- by counting your pulse for 60 seconds

Lower resting heart rates often reflect better cardiovascular conditioning and recovery.

Glucose

Record your fasting blood glucose.

For the most consistent readings:

• measure first thing in the morning

• measure before eating or drinking anything except water

Record the value shown on your glucose meter.

Example:

92 mg/dL

Sleep

Record the approximate number of hours you slept the previous night.

Example:

7.5 hours

Sleep quality strongly influences many metabolic signals, including glucose levels, blood pressure, and heart rate.

Activity

Write the primary movement or exercise you performed that day.

Examples:

• walk

• strength training

• yoga

• cycling

• rest

Recording the type of activity can help reveal patterns between movement and metabolic health.

Notes

Use this space to record anything that may have influenced your numbers.

Examples:

- late dinner
- stressful day
- illness
- travel
- unusually poor sleep

These notes often help explain changes in your metabolic signals.

Calculating Weekly Averages

At the end of each weekly tracker page, you will see spaces to calculate several averages.

These averages help you observe trends rather than individual daily fluctuations.

Average Weight

Add the weights recorded for the week and divide by 7.

Example:

150 + 149 + 150 + 151 + 149 + 150 + 150 = 1049

1049 ÷ 7 = 149.9

Average Weight = 149.9

Average Fasting Glucose

Add the glucose readings for the week and divide by 7.

This provides a clearer picture of overall glucose trends.

Average Sleep

Add the number of hours slept each night and divide by 7.

This shows your average nightly sleep duration.

Average Resting Heart Rate

Add your daily resting heart rate values and divide by 7.

This can reveal changes in fitness, stress levels, and recovery.

Using the Reflection Questions

After calculating your averages, take a moment to reflect on your week.

Consider questions such as:

- What habits helped improve my numbers this week?
- What factors may have raised my numbers?
- What is one small change I could try next week?

These reflections help turn daily tracking into meaningful insight.

Tools You May Need

Some measurements in this tracker require simple health monitoring tools, such as a digital scale, a measuring tape, a blood pressure monitor, or a blood glucose meter.

If you do not already have these tools, they are widely available and easy to obtain. Most pharmacies, drug stores, and major retailers such as Walmart, Target, and many grocery stores carry them in their health sections. They can also be purchased through many online retailers.

Many affordable home blood pressure monitors and glucose meters are designed specifically for personal use and include clear instructions for accurate measurements.

If you choose not to track certain metrics, you may simply leave those fields blank and focus on the signals you are able to record.

Helpful Tools for Tracking

• Digital body weight scale

• Flexible measuring tape

• Home blood pressure monitor

• Blood glucose meter

• Notebook or pen

Your 90-Day Starting Point

Before beginning your daily tracking, take a moment to record your starting measurements. These numbers will serve as a reference point so that you can observe how your metabolic signals change over the next ninety days.

Baseline Measurement Table

Metric	Starting Value
Date	
Weight	
Waist Circumference	
Blood Pressure	
Resting Heart Rate	
Fasting Glucose	
Avg Sleep (past week)	
Typical Daily Activity Level	

Current Habits Snapshot

How many days per week do you currently exercise?

____

Typical Bedtime:

____

Typical dinner time:

____

Anything else you want to remember about your current habits:

____

____

These starting values are simply a snapshot of where you are today. Over the next ninety days, your daily entries will help reveal patterns and progress that may not be visible day to day.

Metabolic Tracking Pages

Week ________________________

Date	Weight	Waist (in.)	Blood Pressure	Heart Rate	Glucose (AM)	Sleep (Hrs.)	Exercise/ Activity	Notes

---

Weekly Reflection:

Average Weight: ____________
Average Fasting Glucose: ____________
Average Sleep: ____________
Energy Level (1-10): ____________

Reflection Questions:

What habits helped my numbers this week?

____

What habits may have raised my numbers?

____

What is one small improvement for next week?

____

Week ______________________

Date	Weight	Waist (in.)	Blood Pressure	Heart Rate	Glucose (AM)	Sleep (Hrs.)	Exercise/ Activity	Notes

Weekly Reflection:

Average Weight: __________
Average Fasting Glucose: __________
Average Sleep: __________
Energy Level (1-10): __________

Reflection Questions:

What habits helped my numbers this week?

____

What habits may have raised my numbers?

____

What is one small improvement for next week?

____

Week ______________________

Date	Weight	Waist (in.)	Blood Pressure	Heart Rate	Glucose (AM)	Sleep (Hrs.)	Exercise/ Activity	Notes

Weekly Reflection:

Average Weight: ____________
Average Fasting Glucose: ____________
Average Sleep: ____________
Energy Level (1-10): ____________

Reflection Questions:

What habits helped my numbers this week?

____

What habits may have raised my numbers?

____

What is one small improvement for next week?

____

Week ____________________________

Date	Weight	Waist (in.)	Blood Pressure	Heart Rate	Glucose (AM)	Sleep (Hrs.)	Exercise/ Activity	Notes

Weekly Reflection:

Average Weight: ___________
Average Fasting Glucose: ___________
Average Sleep: ___________
Energy Level (1-10): ___________

Reflection Questions:

What habits helped my numbers this week?

____

What habits may have raised my numbers?

____

What is one small improvement for next week?

____

Week ______________________

Date	Weight	Waist (in.)	Blood Pressure	Heart Rate	Glucose (AM)	Sleep (Hrs.)	Exercise/ Activity	Notes

Weekly Reflection:

Average Weight: __________
Average Fasting Glucose: __________
Average Sleep: __________
Energy Level (1-10): __________

Reflection Questions:

What habits helped my numbers this week?

____

What habits may have raised my numbers?

____

What is one small improvement for next week?

____

Week ______________________

Date	Weight	Waist (in.)	Blood Pressure	Heart Rate	Glucose (AM)	Sleep (Hrs.)	Exercise/ Activity	Notes

Weekly Reflection:

Average Weight: __________
Average Fasting Glucose: __________
Average Sleep: __________
Energy Level (1-10): __________

Reflection Questions:

What habits helped my numbers this week?

____

What habits may have raised my numbers?

____

What is one small improvement for next week?

____

Week ____________________________

Date	Weight	Waist (in.)	Blood Pressure	Heart Rate	Glucose (AM)	Sleep (Hrs.)	Exercise/ Activity	Notes

---

Weekly Reflection:

Average Weight: ____________
Average Fasting Glucose: ____________
Average Sleep: ____________
Energy Level (1-10): ____________

Reflection Questions:

What habits helped my numbers this week?

____

What habits may have raised my numbers?

____

What is one small improvement for next week?

____

Week ______________________

Date	Weight	Waist (in.)	Blood Pressure	Heart Rate	Glucose (AM)	Sleep (Hrs.)	Exercise/ Activity	Notes

Weekly Reflection:

Average Weight: ___________
Average Fasting Glucose: ___________
Average Sleep: ___________
Energy Level (1-10): ___________

Reflection Questions:

What habits helped my numbers this week?

____

What habits may have raised my numbers?

____

What is one small improvement for next week?

____

Week ______________________

Date	Weight	Waist (in.)	Blood Pressure	Heart Rate	Glucose (AM)	Sleep (Hrs.)	Exercise/ Activity	Notes

Weekly Reflection:

Average Weight: ____________
Average Fasting Glucose: ____________
Average Sleep: ____________
Energy Level (1-10): ____________

Reflection Questions:

What habits helped my numbers this week?

____

What habits may have raised my numbers?

____

What is one small improvement for next week?

____

Week ______________________

Date	Weight	Waist (in.)	Blood Pressure	Heart Rate	Glucose (AM)	Sleep (Hrs.)	Exercise/ Activity	Notes

---

Weekly Reflection:

Average Weight: __________
Average Fasting Glucose: __________
Average Sleep: __________
Energy Level (1-10): __________

Reflection Questions:

What habits helped my numbers this week?

____

What habits may have raised my numbers?

____

What is one small improvement for next week?

____

Week ____________________

Date	Weight	Waist (in.)	Blood Pressure	Heart Rate	Glucose (AM)	Sleep (Hrs.)	Exercise/ Activity	Notes

Weekly Reflection:

Average Weight: ____________
Average Fasting Glucose: ____________
Average Sleep: ____________
Energy Level (1-10): ____________

Reflection Questions:

What habits helped my numbers this week?

____

What habits may have raised my numbers?

____

What is one small improvement for next week?

____

Week ______________________

Date	Weight	Waist (in.)	Blood Pressure	Heart Rate	Glucose (AM)	Sleep (Hrs.)	Exercise/ Activity	Notes

Weekly Reflection:

Average Weight: ____________
Average Fasting Glucose: ____________
Average Sleep: ____________
Energy Level (1-10): ____________

Reflection Questions:

What habits helped my numbers this week?

____

What habits may have raised my numbers?

____

What is one small improvement for next week?

____

Week ______________________

Date	Weight	Waist (in.)	Blood Pressure	Heart Rate	Glucose (AM)	Sleep (Hrs.)	Exercise/ Activity	Notes

Weekly Reflection:

Average Weight: __________
Average Fasting Glucose: __________
Average Sleep: __________
Energy Level (1-10): __________

Reflection Questions:

What habits helped my numbers this week?

____

What habits may have raised my numbers?

____

What is one small improvement for next week?

____

Your 90-Day Results

Metric	Starting Value	Current Value	Change
Weight			
Waist			
Blood Pressure			
Resting Heart Rate			
Fasting Glucose			
Average Sleep			

What improvements did you notice?

____

What habits helped the most?

____

What changes will you continue?

____

Understanding the Patterns You May See

Over ninety days of tracking, many people begin to notice patterns in their metabolic signals. These patterns can provide clues about how sleep, activity, stress, and meal timing affect the body.

The patterns you observe are not diagnoses. Instead, they are useful signals that can help guide small adjustments in daily habits.

Some patterns are encouraging. Others may suggest that certain habits are working against you. Not every unusual number means something serious, but repeated trends can offer useful clues. Minor factors such as poor sleep, dehydration, late meals, emotional stress, illness, travel, changes in routine, or inactivity may affect your readings. If a concerning pattern continues or worsens, it is wise to discuss it with a qualified healthcare professional.

Patterns become useful when they lead to small experiments. If you notice the same trend repeatedly, try changing one variable at a time — such as dinner timing, sleep routine, walking after meals, hydration, or daily movement — and observe whether your numbers respond. Small, consistent changes are often easier to evaluate than trying to change everything at once.

Below are a few common patterns people often notice while tracking metabolic health:

Pattern 1 — Morning Glucose Is Higher After Late Dinners

What it might mean:

When meals are eaten late in the evening, the body may still be processing glucose during the night. This can sometimes lead to higher fasting glucose readings in the morning.

Possible adjustments:

• Finish dinner earlier when possible

• Reduce late-night snacking

• Try a short walk after dinner

Pattern 2 — Resting Heart Rate Is Higher After Poor Sleep

What it might mean:

Sleep plays a critical role in recovery and nervous system balance. Poor sleep often raises resting heart rate and may also influence blood pressure and glucose levels.

Possible adjustments:

• Aim for consistent bedtimes

• Reduce screen exposure before sleep

• Create a calming bedtime routine

Pattern 3 — Weight Fluctuates but Waist Measurement Changes Slowly

What it might mean:

Body weight naturally fluctuates from day to day due to hydration, food intake, and other factors. Waist measurements often change more slowly and may better reflect longer-term body composition changes.

Possible adjustments:

• Focus on weekly trends instead of daily weight

• Maintain consistent physical activity

• Prioritize whole foods

Pattern 4 — Blood Pressure Improves With Regular Activity

What it might mean:

Regular movement supports cardiovascular health. Even moderate daily activity can influence blood pressure readings over time.

Possible adjustments:

• Add short walks during the day

• Aim for consistent weekly movement

• Reduce long periods of sitting

Pattern 5 — Better Sleep Improves Multiple Numbers

What it might mean:

Sleep affects many metabolic systems. Improvements in sleep often influence resting heart rate, glucose regulation, and overall energy levels.

Possible adjustments:

- Prioritize consistent sleep duration
- Maintain a regular bedtime routine
- Limit caffeine later in the day

Tracking metabolic signals helps reveal how the body responds to daily habits. The patterns you observe are not meant to create pressure or perfection. Instead, they offer helpful information that can guide small adjustments over time.

Even modest changes in sleep, activity, and daily routines can gradually support a healthier metabolic balance.

Common Unhelpful Patterns to Watch For

Fasting glucose stays elevated for several mornings in a row

Possible minor causes: late dinners, poor sleep, stress, illness, less activity than usual, or more refined carbohydrates.

What to try: earlier dinners, a short walk after dinner, better sleep consistency, improved hydration, and reviewing evening food choices.

Blood pressure is higher on stressful or poorly rested days

Possible minor causes: stress, inadequate sleep, dehydration, excess sodium, pain, or caffeine close to measurement time.

What to try: measure after sitting quietly, improve hydration, track sleep, and recheck under calmer conditions.

Resting heart rate trends upward over several days

Possible minor causes: poor sleep, stress, dehydration, illness, overexertion, or reduced recovery.

What to try: prioritize rest, hydrate, and note whether you may be getting sick or are under unusual strain.

Weight jumps quickly over a day or two

Possible minor causes: water retention, salty foods, hormonal shifts, constipation, travel, or later meals.

What to try: focus on weekly averages rather than one day, and look for repeat trends instead of reacting to a single reading.

Continuing Your Metabolic Health Journey

Over the past ninety days, you have taken an important step toward understanding how your body responds to your daily habits.

By recording your metabolic signals consistently, you may have noticed patterns in how sleep, activity, stress, meal timing, and other factors influence your numbers.

These observations are valuable.

Metabolic health is not determined by a single number or a single moment. It reflects patterns that develop over time. The awareness you gained during this process can help guide your decisions moving forward.

Some people choose to continue tracking beyond ninety days, beginning a new cycle of observation and reflection. Others use what they learned to focus on a few key habits that produced the most positive changes.

There is no single correct approach.

The most important outcome of this process is the understanding you gained about your own body.

Small, consistent habits often lead to the most meaningful improvements over time.

Using What You Learned

After ninety days of tracking, many people discover that their metabolic signals respond strongly to a few specific habits. The goal of this workbook is not simply to collect numbers, but to help you identify which daily behaviors most influence your health.

You may notice that certain adjustments consistently improve your readings. For example:

• finishing dinner earlier

• walking after meals

• improving sleep consistency

• increasing daily movement

• reducing highly processed foods

• improving hydration

When you identify patterns like these, you can begin making small, intentional adjustments.

Rather than trying to change everything at once, choose **one or two habits** to improve and observe how your body responds over the following weeks.

Many people find that once they understand their personal patterns, maintaining metabolic health becomes much easier. Instead of guessing, they can rely on the signals their body provides.

The numbers you tracked are simply tools. The real value lies in the awareness they helped you build.

Made in the USA
Monee, IL
10 November 2026

68380050R00022